The Fibromyalgia Cookbook

A Hands-on Guide to Essential Food Selection for Pain Reduction and Improved Health.

Michael Murray

CONTENT

INTRODUCTION

The Introduction to The Fibromyalgia Cookbook. Bringing to Light the Regenerative Potential of Food for Energy and Pain Management.

Welcome to a trip where the kitchen becomes a refuge and every ingredient has the power to provide comfort and refreshment. Together, using "The Fibromyalgia Cookbook," we embarked on a transformative adventure exploring the world of nutritious, fibromyalgia-friendly food. It is a guide, a companion, and proof of the undeniable link between our mental and physical well-being.

These sections provide meals and well-being strategies in addition to recipes and lots of attention. By means of this culinary exploration, we will uncover the astounding potential of thoughtful food choices to reduce discomfort, boost energy, and restore balance in spite of the challenges posed by fibromyalgia.

All of the dishes showcase the healing potential of wholesome, fibromyalgia-friendly foods: from vibrant platters of nutrient-dense meals that arouse the senses to comforting soups that uplift the soul.

But it's more than just an assortment of delectable dishes. Here, too, we'll learn about the health advantages of herbs and spices, explore how easy meal preparation is, and develop a clever, considerate grocery shopping and menu planning strategy. Together, we'll prepare not only meals but also cozy, resilient, and joyful moments.

Thus, "The Fibromyalgia Cookbook" is your trustworthy companion whether you're seeking nourishment while dealing with discomfort, striving for energy in your daily life, or just want the pleasure of consuming foods that are beneficial to your health.

I hope these pages serve as a haven, your go-to resource for recipe ideas, and the beginning of a journey towards improved enjoyment and health. Let's recognise the ability of food to transform lives, one delectable and nourishing bite at a time.

Join us as we go on a delightful adventure to improve our health, lessen discomfort, and rekindle our passion for life.

Chapter 1: Understanding Nutrition and Fibromyalgia

In the realm of fibromyalgia, where symptom treatment involves both art and science, nutrition is essential for potential relief and revitalization. Understanding how food impacts the body and how that influences fibromyalgia symptoms is essential to empowering well-being. In this first chapter, we will delve into the intricate link between food and fibromyalgia, addressing the key concepts and laying the groundwork for a possibly healing dietary journey.

- Diet's Impact on Fibromyalgia Symptoms

Maintaining a conscious, dietary regimen suitable for fibromyalgia is crucial for symptom management and overall health enhancement. Recent studies suggest that eating choices may have a significant impact on the fatigue, chronic pain, and cognitive deficits associated with fibromyalgia.

For instance, a 2021 study examined how a low-FODMAPS diet affected fibromyalgia symptoms, and it was published in the "Clinical Rheumatology" journal. The findings demonstrated a reduction in the participants' pain and other symptoms, suggesting a potential role for dietary intervention in the treatment of fibromyalgia-related discomfort.

- Nutritional Principles That Are Fibromyalgia-Friendly

Anti-Inflammatory Diets: The Foundation of Solace

Inflammation is a common feature of fibromyalgia, exacerbating pain and other symptoms. You might incorporate meals that reduce inflammation to mitigate this effect. This dish serves as an example of how to use anti-inflammatory foods:

Recipe:Anti-Inflammatory **Turmeric-Ginger Smoothie**
- Elements:
- One cup of your preferred milk alternative, such as coconut milk
- One fully grown banana
- One-half tsp ground turmeric
- Grate half a teaspoon of fresh ginger
1/3 cup of chia seeds
- If preferred, one tablespoon of honey
- 1/2 cup of frozen pineapple chunks
- Prepare:
- Use a blender to combine all of the ingredients.
- Blend until smooth and creamy.
- Thank You:
Savour the smoothie's strong anti-inflammatory qualities after pouring it into a glass.

- Foods High in Nutrients: Crucial for Sustaining Energy Over Time

For those with fibromyalgia in particular, maintaining energy and minimising fatigue are crucial aspects of a healthy diet.

This recipe is an example of how to make use of nutrient-dense options:

Recipe: **Quinoa and Black Bean Salad**

- Elements:
- One cup cooked quinoa
One can of black beans, rinsed and drained
- One red bell pepper, cut
- Half a cup of chopped cucumbers
- 1/4 cup finely cut cilantro, just now
- 14 ounces of extra virgin olive oil
- Freshly squeezed lime juice, two teaspoons
- A teaspoon of powdered cumin
Add salt and pepper to taste.

- Prepare:

- In a large bowl, mix the quinoa, black beans, bell pepper, cucumber, and cilantro.
- In a separate small dish, mix the cumin, lime juice, and olive oil. For seasoning, add salt and pepper.
- Pour the dressing over the quinoa mixture and well combine.

- Serve:
Savour this vibrant, high-protein salad as an appetiser or main meal to get a burst of nutrients.

Conclusion, A culinary Empowerment autonomy

I hope these recipes and examples will inspire you to learn more about the connection between nutrition and fibromyalgia and will demonstrate the remarkable role food plays in both boosting health and easing the symptoms of the condition. In the next chapters, we'll delve into more diverse recipes, all of which have been carefully chosen to enhance food's transformative power and provide a satisfying escape from suffering.

By incorporating these fibromyalgia-friendly recipes into your regular cooking routine, you're not only taking care of your health but also opening the door to a life of culinary empowerment, symptom relief, and the profound satisfaction that comes from consuming foods that are supposed to uplift and calm.

Chapter 2: Building a Fibromyalgia-Friendly Pantry

A well-stocked pantry full of foods that are good for fibromyalgia sufferers should be the cornerstone of your kitchen haven. Here is where nutritious, vibrant food grows and flourishes. The foundations covered in this chapter will ensure that your pantry is a veritable haven, brimming with a vast array of goods that form the foundation of soothing, anti-inflammatory, and nutritious dishes.

Accepting Decisions That Don't Inflame

Inflammation is a common enemy in the tale of fibromyalgia, causing constant agony and suffering for those who experience it. When preparing meals that both stimulate and relieve pain, it is imperative to give non-inflammatory ingredients first priority.

- Healthful Grains and Vegetables

1. Quinoa: This gluten-free, nutrient-dense seed works well as a versatile base for salads, grain bowls, and pilafs. It also offers an excellent amount of protein and essential amino acids.

2. Black beans: Packed in antioxidants, fibre, and protein, black beans give a lot of nutrients and body to soups, salads, and major vegetarian entrees.

- Options for Vitamin-Rich Comfort

Vitamins are essential for sustaining bodily functions and energy levels. Your pantry serves as the base for incorporating essential nutrients into your meals.

- The Bright Profusion of Fruits and Vegetables

1. Rich in vitamins A and K, spinach may be cooked in a number of ways, including as a wholesome base for salads, smoothies, and sautés of vegetables.

2. Blueberries: Rich in antioxidants and vitamin C, blueberries provide flavour and nutrition to breakfast dishes, desserts, and snacks.

- Constructing a Practical and Healing Pantry

- Flexible Bases to Fit a Range of Dishes

1. Canned Tomatoes: A staple in stews, soups, and sauces, canned tomatoes are the foundation of a lot of comforting, healthful meals that are appropriate for fibromyalgia sufferers.

2. Brown Rice: Packed with fibre and packed with essential nutrients, brown rice is a hearty and satisfying alternative to refined grains. It makes a great foundation for meals such as stir-fries and pilafs.

- Helpful Tips for Keeping Pantries Organised and Maintained

- Sorting and Labelling to Increase Output

Consider labelling and organising the items in your pantry to provide convenient access and effective inventory control. To make meal preparation simple and enjoyable, create distinct spaces for oils, canned goods, cereals, and beans.

- Keeping an eye on expiry dates

Regularly check the items in your pantry, being mindful of any expiration dates. Throw away any expired foods to maintain your ingredients robust, fresh, and ready for culinary creativity.

- Concluding Remarks: An Introduction to Culinary Adventures

Keeping a well-stocked pantry full of fibromyalgia-friendly foods is more than simply organising supplies; it's a gateway to a world of culinary options full of nourishing snacks, energetic dinners, and comforting treats that are all designed to reduce symptoms and improve your overall health. We'll make the most of these staple components by preparing tasty, anti-inflammatory meals in the next chapters. We'll guide you through practical methods and wholesome dishes that will quickly become favourites in your recipe collection for people with fibromyalgia.

Chapter 3: Harmonious Energy via Satisfying Mornings

Breakfast is the start of opportunity, giving each day vitality and nourishment. With healthy comfort food and well-balanced energy, these breakfast options for people with fibromyalgia may energise your morning and fortify your day. This chapter takes you on a tour of a few of them.

- The Promise of Nourishment at Dawn

A hearty, balanced breakfast lays the foundation for a successful day. It could also provide fibromyalgia sufferers sustained energy levels and symptom alleviation.

- **Muesli**: A Morning Sanctuary Rich in Nutrients

Recipe : **Nutty Muesli Bowl**

- Elements:
- One-half cup steel-cut oats

- One cup of your favourite milk or water

1/3 cup of chia seeds

- 1/4 cup of almond, walnut, or pecan pieces chopped

- One tsp honey or maple syrup

A sprinkle of cinnamon

- Prepare:

- In a saucepan, bring the milk or water to a boil. Stir in the oats and chia seeds.

Reduce the heat and cook the oats, stirring occasionally, for five to seven minutes, or until they reach the desired consistency.

- Spoon the muesli into a bowl and top with chopped almonds, cinnamon, and a honey or syrup drizzle.

Savour this hearty and comforting morning meal.

Because of its critical nutrients and creamy texture, muesli is a comforting and fibromyalgia-friendly breakfast choice. Thanks to the added protein, fibre, and omega-3 fatty acids from the chia seeds, this is a nutrient-dense and energetic meal.

Hearty Quinoa for Morning

Recipe: **Apple Cinnamon Quinoa Porridge**

- Elements:
- 1/2 cup of quinoa
- One cup of your favourite milk or water
- One apple, cored, cut, and peeled
- 1/4 teaspoon of cinnamon powder
- If preferred, add one tablespoon of chopped nuts.
- One tsp honey or maple syrup
- Prepare:
- Rinse the quinoa with a little water.
- In a saucepan, combine the quinoa, milk or water, and apple slices. Bring to a boil.
- Cover the saucepan and simmer the quinoa over low heat for 15 to 20 minutes, or until it is tender and the liquid has been absorbed. Stir in the syrup (or honey) and cinnamon. If preferred, sprinkle chopped nuts over the porridge that is served in bowls.

Rich in essential nutrients and appropriate for fibromyalgia sufferers, this quinoa porridge is a comforting, warm breakfast choice that mixes the subtle sweetness of apple with the comforting effect of cinnamon.

- Incorporating Healthful Twists into Timeless Favourites

- Fruit and Yoghurt Parfait: An Intense and Energising Blend

Recipe: **Berry Yoghurt Parfait**
- Elements:
- A single Greek yoghurt cup
- A half-cup of berries combined with strawberries, blueberries, and raspberries
One-fourth cup granola
A single teaspoon of honey or agave nectar
- Prepare:
- Layer the Greek yoghurt, mixed berries, and granola in a glass.

- Drizzle some honey or agave nectar over top to add a touch of sweetness.
Savour this energising, high-protein breakfast meal.

A vibrant and fibromyalgia-friendly way to start the day is with a fruit and yoghurt parfait, which offers a wonderful burst of colour, vitamins, and protein.

- Final Thoughts: Embracing Satisfying Morning Routines

When you include these fibromyalgia-friendly breakfast recipes into your daily routine, you're not only promoting your health but also ringing in a new day full of comfort and vitality. The promise of nourishment before dawn, which alludes to the potential for mild symptom alleviation, extended vigour, and a deep sense of well-being, sets sail on a journey of balanced health and culinary delight.

In the next chapters, we'll continue to explore a wide range of fibromyalgia-friendly recipes, guiding you through practical methods and positive culinary creations meant to improve your health and provide gratifying pain relief.

Chapter 4: Comforting Soups and Stews

A favourite among fibromyalgia-friendly food ideas are soups and stews, which provide a delicious symphony of tastes and are quite easy to prepare. This chapter takes us on a journey through a variety of nourishing and soothing dishes that all follow the principles of eating well with fibromyalgia.

- The Craft of Comfort and Wholeness

Soups and stews, with their velvety embrace of minerals and calming tastes, provide an opportunity to nourish the body and transform simple ingredients into a harmonious blend of health and energy.

Creating Flavour and Nourishment with Hearty Vegetable Soups

Recipe: Boost Immunity with Vegetable Broth

- Elements:
Eight water cups
- Dice two carrots slightly.
- Two celery stalks cut thinly.
- One onion, quartered
- Four cloves of smashed garlic
- A freshly chopped 1-inch piece of ginger
- A teaspoon of whole black peppercorns
- Two bay leaves
- Prepare:
- Fill a large pot with all the ingredients. Reduce the heat and simmer the mixture for one to two hours after bringing it to a boil.
- Strain the broth using a fine-mesh strainer, discarding the solids.
- Your homemade vegetable broth is ready to use as a tasty and nourishing foundation for a wide range of soups and stews. It also strengthens immunity.

Recipe: Lentil and Vegetable Stew

- Elements:
A cup of rinsed brown or green lentils
– Four cups vegetable-based broth
- Two carrots, chopped
- Two celery stalks, chopped
- A single onion, chopped
- Three cloves of minced garlic
- A teaspoon of powdered cumin
- One teaspoon smoky paprika
Add salt and pepper to taste.
- Prepare:
In a large saucepan, add the lentils, vegetable broth, carrots, celery, onion, and garlic.

Add the cumin and paprika. Once the stew to a boil, reduce the heat and simmer it until the lentils and vegetables are tender, 25 to 30 minutes.

- Season with salt and pepper, to taste. Enjoy this substantial and satisfying lentil stew.

- Including Stems Packed with Protein to Promote Tenderness

- Savouring the Cosiness of Chicken and Vegetable Soup

Recipe: Chicken and Vegetable Soup

- Elements:

A cup and a half of chicken stock

1 A cup of cooked, shredded chicken

- Two carrots, cut
- Two celery stalks, chopped
- A single onion, chopped
- Two cloves of minced garlic
- One teaspoon of dried thyme
- A half-cup of quinoa or uncooked rice
- Prepare:
- In a saucepan, bring the chicken stock to a boil. Add the carrots, celery, onion, garlic, and thyme and stir.
- Simmer the vegetables until they are tender, 15 to 20 minutes.

- Include the cooked chicken together with the rice or quinoa. Simmer for a further 15 to 20 minutes, or until the rice or quinoa is well cooked.

Savour this hearty, high-protein soup prepared with chicken and veggies.

Warm Barley Stew with Beef: A Cosy and Rustic Friend

Recipe: **Barley and Beef Stew** Elements:

- A one pound of stew beef cubes

Four cups of meat-based broth.

- A single onion, chopped
- Two carrots, cut
- Two celery stalks, chopped
– One cup of barley pearls
- Two cloves of minced garlic

A teaspoon of dehydrated rosemary

Add salt and pepper to taste.

- Prepare:
- In a Dutch oven, brown the beef over medium-high heat.

- Include the onion, celery, carrots, and garlic. Cook the vegetables until they start to go soft.
- Pour in the beef broth and then add the barley and rosemary.
- Simmer over low heat for 1 to 2 hours, or until the meat is tender and the barley is fully cooked.
This is a fibromyalgia-friendly stew made with beef and barley that will warm and support you.

Concluding Remarks: An Ode to Harmonious Cosiness

Soups and other dietary choices that are beneficial for fibromyalgia

Stews sing, a combination of nourishment and warmth. By making these meals, you may relieve the pain and discomfort caused by fibromyalgia while also giving your body the essential nutrients and calming tastes. In the next chapters, we'll carry out more of the food inquiry, guiding you through practical tips and a range of happy meals that are said to improve wellness and provide satisfying pain relief.

Chapter 5: Reviving Salads and Lunch Bowls with a Bright Midday Symphony

Lunch is an important meal break because it gives you a time to relax and refuel your body with a vibrant array of nutrients. This chapter explores the world of healthy lunch options that are suitable for people with fibromyalgia, including a range of salad and bowl dishes that will stimulate your senses and enhance your general well-being.

- Acknowledging the Dream of Fullness

Lunchtime salads and bowls provide an abundance of colours, textures, and flavours that blend to produce a lively, nourishing tune that complements the core principles of fibromyalgia-friendly nutrition.

- Preparing a Plant-Powered Grain Bowl Lunch

Recipe: **A dish of quinoa with Mediterranean flavours**

- Elements:
- One cup cooked quinoa
One cup of chickpeas, drained and rinsed
- Chopped half of a cucumber
- A half-cup of tomatoes with seeds
- 1/4 cup of Kalamata olives, pitted and sliced
- 1/4 cup of crumbled feta cheese
- Prepare:
- In a bowl, mix the quinoa, chickpeas, olives, tomatoes, and cucumber.
Top with a little feta cheese crumbles.
- Drizzle with lemon vinaigrette or your preferred dressing.
Enjoy this vibrant and invigorating Mediterranean quinoa dish.

- Vegetable Delight with Rich and Nutritious Salad Bowls

Recipe: **Rainbow Veggie Salad Bowl with Turmeric Dressing**

- Elements:
- Four cups mixed greens, including rocket, spinach, and kale
- One cup of finely chopped red cabbage
- Half a cup of shredded carrots
- Chopped bell peppers, either orange, yellow, or red, about 1/2 cup
- 1/4 cup of quinoa, cooked and cooled
A quarter cup of seeds from sunflowers
- Turmeric dressing:
- 14 ounces of extra virgin olive oil
- Two tablespoons of apple cider vinegar
1 A single teaspoon of dijon mustard
- One teaspoon of turmeric powder
Add salt and pepper to taste.
- Prepare:
- Fill a bowl with the quinoa, mixed greens, bell peppers, carrots, and red cabbage.
- Sprinkle on some sunflower seeds.

- Process all the ingredients for the turmeric vinaigrette in a blender, then transfer to the salad.

Savour the rainbow of hues and an abundance of nutrients in this salad meal made of vegetables.

- Infusing Protein-Packed Creations into Life

Grilled chicken salads' capacity to fill you up

Recipe: **Avocado and Grilled Chicken Salad**

-Elements:

- A double-cup of mixed green salad
- One grilled chicken breast, sliced
- Cut avocado in half
- 1/4 cup of cherry tomatoes cut in half
- 1/4 cup of cucumber slices
— A double-stick of balsamic vinaigrette
- Prepare:

Arrange mixed greens in a salad plate.

- Top with grilled chicken, cherry tomatoes, cucumbers, and avocado.
- Drizzle with balsamic vinaigrette or your preferred dressing.
Enjoy the filling, high-protein hug of this meal of grilled chicken and avocado salad.

- Adopting a Quinoa and Chickpea Salad to Encourage Wholesome Plants

Recipe: Quinoa and Chickpea Power Salad

- Elements:
- Two cups cooked quinoa
A one can of rinsed and drained lentils
- Chopped half a cup of red bell pepper
1/4 cup finely chopped red onion
One-fourth cup of finely chopped parsley
- Two tablespoons of olive oil
- One-half cup of juiced lemon
Add salt and pepper to taste.
- Prepare:
- In a bowl, mix the quinoa, chickpeas, red bell pepper, red onion, and parsley.

- Drizzle the salad with the lemon juice and olive oil mixture.
Toss again after adding salt and pepper to taste.
Savour the plant-based, nutrient-dense core of this quinoa and chickpea power salad.

Final Thoughts: A Symphony of Midday Eats

You may provide your body the essential nutrients and tasty sustenance it needs during your noon break by including these fibromyalgia-friendly salad and lunch bowl meals. It also gives you a respite from the grind.

bringing vitality and lots of reassurance into your day. Next, we'll go further into a range of fibromyalgia-friendly recipes, guiding you through realistic approaches and a colourful mosaic of inspired dishes meant to improve health and provide revitalising nutrition.

Chapter 5: Potent Salads and Bowls for Lunch

Chapter 5 turns into a haven for those searching for nourishment in the vibrant world of fibromyalgia-friendly food or for an energy boost to get through the day. "Energising Lunch Bowls and Salads" offers a symphony of flavours and nutrients that have been carefully selected to boost energy and satisfy the particular needs of fibromyalgia sufferers.

- Synopsis of Bright Energy

Due to our busy schedules, taking a nourishing and revitalising lunch break becomes crucial self-care. This chapter is a tribute to vibrant, nutrient-dense salads and bowls that satisfy the body's needs all day long and arouse the senses.

The first dish is a **QUINOA AND ROASTED VEGGIE POWER BOWL**

Recipe

• A cup of washed and cooked quinoa

• A single sweet potato, chopped

• A single, sliced courgette

• One red bell pepper, chopped

• Cherry tomatoes, halved

• A pair of tablespoons olive oil

• Add pepper and salt to taste.

• 1/4 cup of hummus (to serve)

Getting ready:

Put the oven on to 200°C, or 400°F.

• Toss the sweet potato, zucchini and red pepper with the olive oil, salt and pepper.

• Bake the vegetables for twenty to twenty-five minutes, until they are tender and starting to become caramelised.

• To build the dish, add the roasted vegetables on top and the cooked quinoa on bottom.

• Add a spoonful of hummus for a creamy finish.

Recipe 2: **Chickpeas and Spinach with Citrus Salad**

Elements:

• Four glasses of fresh spinach

• Fifteen ounces (one can) of rinsed and drained chickpeas

• One peeled and split orange

• Thinly chop a red onion in half

• 1/4 cup of sliced almonds

• A pair of tablespoons olive oil

• 10 milligrammes of vinegar with balsamic flavour

• Add pepper and salt to taste.

Getting ready:

In a large bowl, mix together the chickpeas, sliced almonds, orange segments, red onion, and fresh spinach.

• In a small bowl, mix the olive oil, balsamic vinegar, salt, and pepper to create the dressing.

• Drizzle with the salad dressing and mix to coat.

• Serve immediately for a tangy, energising boost.

Recipe: **A bowl of Mediterranean quinoa salad is the third.**

Elements:

• A single cup of cold, cooked quinoa

• One cucumber, diced

• Cherry tomatoes, halved

• Slicing half a cup of Kalamata olives

• 1/4 cup red onion, diced coarsely

• Crushed feta cheese, about half a cup

• Fresh parsley, finely chopped (for garnish)

Putting on clothes:

• Three tsp finely ground olive oil

• Half a teaspoon red wine vinegar

• One teaspoon of dried oregano

• Add pepper and salt to taste.

Getting ready:

• In a large bowl, mix the cooked quinoa, cherry tomatoes, cucumber, red onion, feta cheese, and Kalamata olives.

In a small bowl, mix together the olive oil, red wine vinegar, dried oregano, salt, and pepper to create the dressing.

• Pour the dressing over the quinoa mixture and toss to fully incorporate.

• Enjoy this Mediterranean-inspired meal with a garnish of fresh parsley.

Recipe: **Asian-Inspired Sesame Tofu Salad**

Elements:

• A single block of firm tofu, chopped and pressed

• Four cups salad-worthy mixed greens

• A single carrot, julienned

• One bell pepper, cut into thin slices (any colour)

• Two green onions, chopped

Garnish with sesame seeds

Dressing with ginger seeds:

• One tablespoon soy sauce

• One tablespoon rice vinegar

• TWO SESAMIOL TABLETS

• A tsp of maple syrup

• A teaspoon of finely grated ginger

• One clove of finely chopped garlic

Getting ready:

• In a skillet, fry the cubed tofu until golden brown.

• In a large bowl, mix together the sliced bell pepper, green onions, julienned carrot, and mixed salad greens.

• Combine the soy sauce, rice vinegar, sesame oil, maple syrup, grated ginger, and chopped garlic to create the dressing.

• Gently toss in the sesame ginger dressing and tofu that has been sautéed before adding it to the salad.

• Sprinkle sesame seeds on top for a delightful crunch.

To sum up:

"Energising Lunch Bowls and Salads" transforms lunch into a fine dining experience that offers a burst of flavours and textures along with a rapid energy surge. All of the meals—from the hearty Quinoa and Roasted Vegetable Power Bowl to the refreshing Spinach and Chickpea Citrus Salad—support the notion that eating well can still be tasty and enjoyable, even for those who have fibromyalgia. Accept these vibrant treats and allow each bite to revitalise your body and spirit.

Chapter 6: Mouthwatering Snacks & Appetisers

This Chapter takes readers on a culinary adventure that includes creative and delicious snacks and appetisers with regard to fibromyalgia health and wellbeing. These meals are intended to promote overall health and wellbeing while providing a delightful balance of flavour and nutrition, making them more than just snacks.

Summary of Fibromyalgia-Friendly Snacking

This chapter focuses on snacking, acknowledging that energy levels should be maintained and that fibromyalgia sufferers have specific dietary needs. Each dish demonstrates that snacks don't have to be unhealthy to be decadent, thanks to their nutrient-dense ingredients and careful preparation.

Recipe: **Avocado and white bean dip**

Elements:

• One fifteen-ounce can of white beans, rinsed and drained

• One fully grown avocado, seeded and unseeded

• Freshly squeezed lemon juice, two teaspoons

• Two cloves of minced garlic

• A pair of tablespoons olive oil

• Add pepper and salt to taste.

• Decorating with fresh herbs

Getting ready:

• In a food processor, combine the avocado, white beans, lemon juice, and minced garlic.

• Blend until smooth, adding olive oil a little at a time to get the right consistency.

• Add pepper and salt according to taste.

• Spoon the dip onto a plate, cover with fresh herbs, and serve with whole-grain crackers or sliced vegetables.

Recipe: Stuffed Mushrooms with Quinoa and Veggies

Elements:

• One cup cooked quinoa

• Eight huge mushrooms, with the stems taken off and chopped finely

• Half a cup of roughly chopped red bell pepper

• Half a cup of finely chopped courgette

• 1/4 cup red onion, diced coarsely

• Two cloves of minced garlic

• A teaspoon of thyme, dried

• Half a cup of crumbled feta cheese

• Add pepper and salt to taste.

• Olive oil to use as a drizzle

Getting ready:

• Set oven temperature to 375°F, or 190°C.

• Sauté the red bell pepper, garlic, zucchini, red onion and mushroom stems in a pan until they become soft.

• Put the cooked quinoa, feta cheese, sautéed vegetables, and dried thyme in a bowl. For seasoning, add salt and pepper.

• Once the mushrooms are tender, bake the quinoa mixture in the mushroom caps for 20 to 25 minutes after sprinkling with olive oil.

• Serve these delightful stuffed mushrooms as a filler and appetiser that is ideal for persons with fibromyalgia.

Recipe: **Hummus with spinach and artichokes**

Elements:

• Fifteen ounces (one can) of rinsed and drained chickpeas

• One cup of raw spinach

• One cup of drained artichoke hearts

• One-fourth cup tahini

• Two cloves of minced garlic

• Half a tablespoon of lemon juice

• Three tablespoons of extra virgin olive oil

• Add pepper and salt to taste.

• Vegetable sticks or whole-grain pita bread for dipping

Getting ready:

• Place the chickpeas, spinach, artichoke hearts, tahini, lemon juice, and minced garlic in a food processor.

• Pulse until smooth; add olive oil a bit at a time to reach the desired consistency.

• Add pepper and salt according to taste.

• Spoon the hummus onto a platter and pair it with vegetable sticks or whole-grain pita bread.

Recipe: **Energy Bites with Nuts**

Elements:

• One cup of rolled oats

• A half-cup of almond, peanut, or cashew butter

• 1/4 cup honey or maple syrup

• 1/2 cup ground flaxseeds

• A half-cup of finely chopped nuts, such walnuts, almonds, or pistachios

• 1/4 cup chips made with dark chocolate

• A teaspoon of vanilla extract

• A pinch of salt

Getting ready:

In a large bowl, combine the ground flaxseeds, chopped nuts, chocolate chips, nut butter, vanilla essence, honey or maple syrup, and a pinch of salt.

• Process until well combined.

• Using parchment paper, arrange the bite-sized balls you created from the mixture on a tray.

• Refrigerate the bites for at least 30 minutes to allow them to firm.

These quick and delicious nutty energy nibbles are perfect for anybody with fibromyalgia. Keep them in a container that is sealed.

To sum up

The art of nibbling is transformed into a gourmet festival in Chapter 6, proving that fibromyalgia-friendly food may be both tasty and health-conscious. From decadent dips to savoury stuffed mushrooms and invigorating snacks, each dish showcases the commitment to sating the palate and advancing overall health. You may enjoy the pleasure of mindful eating for those managing their fibromyalgia health and wellness with these tasty and mindfully made candies.

Chapter 7: Main Course Nutrition: Lean Proteins and Plant-Based Treats

Chapter 7, which offers a variety of Nourishing Main Courses that are designed to nourish the body and the mind, is a brilliant example of culinary exploration in the realm of fibromyalgia-friendly meals. These recipes are an explosion of flavour, nutrition, and specifically created support for fibromyalgia patients. They include everything from delectable plant-based foods to lean meats.

Recipe

Plant-Based Treats: Quinoa-Stuffed Acorn Squash

Elements:

• Halved and seeded two acorn squash

• One cup of quinoa, cooked

• A single can (15 ounces) of black beans, washed and drained

• A cup of maize kernels, either fresh or frozen

• Chopped cherry tomatoes in one cup

• One cup of kale, roughly chopped

• A half-cup of red onion, diced finely

• 1/2 cup vegan cheese (optional)

• A teaspoon of powdered cumin

• One teaspoon of powdered chilli

• Add pepper and salt to taste.

• Fresh cilantro for garnish

Getting ready:

Put the oven on to 200°C, or 400°F.

• Arrange the half acorn squash, cut side up, on a baking sheet.

In large bowl, mix cooked quinoa, black beans, corn, kale, red onion, vegan cheese, chilli powder, ground cumin and salt & pepper.

• Stuff the quinoa mixture into the acorn squash on both sides.

• Bake for 25 to 30 minutes, or until the squash is tender.

This colourful, nutrient-dense plant-based main meal may be served by adding some fresh cilantro as a garnish.

Recipe: **Perfectly Packed with Protein: Baked Chicken with Lemon Herbs**

Elements:

• Four chicken breasts deboned and skinless

• A pair of tablespoons olive oil

• Freshly squeezed lemon juice, two teaspoons

• One teaspoon of dried oregano

• One teaspoon dried thyme

• One teaspoon of garlic powder

• Add pepper and salt to taste.

• Lemon slices as a garnish

• Fresh parsley as a garnish

Getting ready:

• Preheat the oven to 375°F, or 190°C.

In a small bowl, mix together the olive oil, lemon juice, thyme, oregano, garlic powder, and pepper.

• Put the chicken breasts in a baking dish and evenly spoon the lemon-herb mixture over them.

• Bake the chicken until it's done, 25 to 30 minutes.

• To make a tasty, high-protein entrée, sprinkle fresh parsley and lemon slices over top before serving.

Recipe: **Harmonious Wholesomeness: Veggies with Stir-fried Lentil**

Elements:

• A cup of prepared green lentils

• Two cups broccoli florets

• One finely sliced red bell pepper

• A single carrot, julienned

• A single, sliced courgette

• One teaspoon of soy sauce with reduced sodium

• TWO SESAMOL TABLETS

• A single teaspoon of rice vinegar.

• A tsp of maple syrup

• Two cloves of minced garlic

• A tsp finely grated ginger

Garnish with sesame seeds

• Add green onions as a garnish

Getting ready:

• In a wok or large pan, warm the sesame oil over medium-high heat.

• Add the broccoli, red pepper, zucchini and carrot. The vegetables should be stir-fried for three to five minutes, or until they begin to soften.

• Add the cooked lentils to the vegetables in the pan.

• In a small bowl, mix together the soy sauce, ginger, garlic, rice vinegar, and maple syrup. Drizzle the sauce over the lentil and vegetable combo.

• Continue to stir-fry for an additional two to three minutes, or until the food is evenly covered in sauce.

• To make a colorful, high-protein plant-based stir-fry, add sesame seeds and green onions as garnish before serving.

Recipe: **Lean and green is the grilled salmon with lemon-dill sauce.**

Elements:

• Four salmon filets

• A pair of tablespoons olive oil

• Freshly squeezed lemon juice, two teaspoons

• One tablespoon of fresh dill, chopped coarsely.

A teaspoon of Dijon mustard

• Add pepper and salt to taste.

• Lemon wedges to serve

• Use fresh dill for garnish.

Getting ready:

• Turn the heat down to medium-high on the grill.

To prepare the sauce, in a small bowl, mix together the olive oil, lemon juice, dill, Dijon mustard, salt, and pepper.

• Drizzle the salmon fillets with sauce on both sides.

• Bake for 4-5 minutes on each side, or until the salmon flakes easily with a fork.

• Serve the grilled salmon with lemon wedges and fresh dill on top as a delicious and low-fat protein choice.

To sum up

In Chapter 7, a culinary tapestry of plant-based marvels and delights high in protein is weaved together to benefit fibromyalgia sufferers. Tasty Main Courses like sizzling grilled salmon and stuffed acorn squash give soothing embraces to please every palette, showcasing the harmonic marriage of taste and wellbeing and proving that delicious meals can be the cornerstone of holistic health. Accept the taste experience and let these recipes be an ode to the joys of conscious, healthful eating.

Chapter 8: Savoury Side Dishes and Pairings

A harmonising group of Flavorful Sides and Accompaniments, Chapter 8 takes centre stage in the culinary symphony of fibromyalgia-friendly meals. Not only can these meals improve your eating experience overall, they also include vital nutrients that enhance general health. Let's look at a range of delectable dishes that will go well with main meals and guarantee a tasty and healthful experience.

Recipe: **Herb-Garlic Roasted Quinoa**

Elements:

• One cup of washed quinoa

• Two cups broth made with vegetables

• One garlic bulb with its cloves removed and peeled

• Two teaspoons of olive oil

• A teaspoon of thyme, dried

• Season with salt and pepper to taste

• As a garnish, fresh parsley

Getting ready:

Start the oven to 400°F, or 200°C.

• Put the quinoa, garlic cloves, vegetable broth, olive oil, thyme, salt, and pepper in a baking dish.

• Bake, covered with foil, for 25 to 30 minutes, or until the garlic is soft and the quinoa is done.

• Use a fork to fluff the quinoa, sprinkle with fresh parsley, and serve as a filling and savoury side dish.

Recipe: **Roasted Vegetables with Turmeric**

Elements:

• Chop various veggies (broccoli, carrots, sweet potatoes, etc.).

• Two teaspoons of olive oil

• One tsp finely ground turmeric

• One teaspoon of cumin

• Season with salt and pepper to taste

• Fresh cilantro for decorating

Getting ready:

Set the oven's temperature to 425°F (220°C).

• Combine the chopped veggies, olive oil, cumin, turmeric, salt, and pepper in a big bowl and toss until well coated.

• Arrange the veggies in a single layer on a baking pan.

• Roast the veggies for 25 to 30 minutes, or until they are soft and golden.

• Add some fresh cilantro as a colourful and nourishing side dish garnish before serving.

Recipe: **Herbed Lemon Quinoa Salad**

Elements:

• One cup cooked and chilled quinoa

• Half a cup of cherry tomatoes

• Diced one cucumber

• 1/4 cup finely chopped red onion

- 1/4 cup finely chopped fresh parsley

- 1/4 cup crumbled feta cheese (optional)

Getting dressed:

- Three tablespoons of extra virgin olive oil

- Half a tablespoon of lemon juice

- One teaspoon of oregano, dried

- Season with salt and pepper to taste

Getting ready:

- Combine quinoa, feta cheese, cucumber, red onion, fresh parsley, and cherry tomatoes in a big bowl.

- To make the dressing, combine the olive oil, lemon juice, dried oregano, salt, and pepper in a small bowl.

• Drizzle the quinoa mixture with the dressing, tossing to thoroughly mix.

• You can have this cool quinoa salad as a light meal or as a side dish.

Recipe: **Balsamic-Glazed Brussels Sprouts**

Elements:

• 1 pound Brussels sprouts, trimmed and halved

• 2 tablespoons balsamic vinegar

• 1 tablespoon olive oil

• 1 tablespoon maple syrup

• Season with salt and pepper to taste

• Crushed red pepper flakes for a hint of heat

Getting ready:

Start the oven to 400°F, or 200°C.

• In a bowl, toss Brussels sprouts with balsamic vinegar, olive oil, maple syrup, salt, and pepper.

• Spread the Brussels sprouts on a baking sheet in a single layer.

• Roast for 20-25 minutes, tossing halfway through, until the sprouts are caramelized and tender.

• Sprinkle with red pepper flakes before serving for a sweet and spicy side dish.

Recipe: **Cumin-Scented Quinoa Pilaf**

Elements:

• One cup of washed quinoa

• Two cups broth made with vegetables

• 1 tablespoon olive oil

• 1 onion, coarsely chopped

• 2 cloves garlic, minced

• 1 teaspoon ground cumin

• 1/2 teaspoon smoked paprika

• Season with salt and pepper to taste

• Fresh cilantro for decorating

Getting ready:

• In a saucepan, heat olive oil over medium heat. Add chopped onion and heat until melted.

• Add minced garlic, ground cumin, smoked paprika, salt, and pepper. Sauté for a further 1-2 minutes.

• Stir in quinoa and simmer for another 2 minutes to toast the grains.

• Pour in vegetable broth, bring to a boil, then decrease heat to low, cover, and simmer for 15-20 minutes or until the quinoa is done.

• Fluff the quinoa with a fork, top with fresh cilantro, and serve as a fragrant and savoury pilaf.

Conclusion

In Chapter 8, Flavorful Sides and Accompaniments become the supporting performers in your fibromyalgia-friendly cooking show. With these recipes, you not only boost the nutritional content of your meals but also add layers of flavour and texture to every mouthful. From roasted veggies to vivid salads, these side dishes are a testimony to the concept that eating healthily can be both tasty and supportive of your health objectives. As you taste these delectable accompaniments, may your dining experience be expanded and your well-being nourished.

Chapter 9: Indulgent-yet-Healthy Desserts

In the realm of fibromyalgia-friendly culinary delights, Chapter 9 emerges as a sweet sanctuary – "Indulgent-yet-Healthy Desserts." Here, we embark on a journey that transcends traditional notions of desserts, introducing a collection of treats that deliver gratifying sweetness while adhering to fibromyalgia-friendly dietary principles.

Introduction: Discovering Delightful Happiness in Health

Desserts are often thought of as indulgence, but when it comes to fibromyalgia, it's important to strike a balance between enjoyment and well-being. This chapter serves as evidence that sweetness does not have to be abandoned and that enjoying delicious foods does not have to come at the expense of wellbeing.

Recipe: **Chocolate Mousse with Avocado**

Elements:

• A pair of mature avocados

• Half a cup of cocoa powder without sugar

• Half a cup of agave nectar or maple syrup

• One tsp vanilla essence

• A little amount of salt

• Ripe berries for garnish

Getting ready:

• Scoop the avocado flesh into a food processor or blender.

• Stir in vanilla essence, maple syrup, cocoa powder, and a little amount of salt.

• Blend until creamy and smooth.

• Refrigerate the mousse for a minimum of 60 minutes.

• For a rich chocolate treat that is suitable for those with fibromyalgia, top with fresh berries and serve.

Recipe: **Energy Bites with Almond Butter**

Elements:

• One cup of rolled oats

• Half a cup of almond butter

• One-third cup maple syrup or honey

• Grounded flaxseeds, 1/2 cup

• Half a cup of coconut, shredded

• One tsp vanilla essence

• Chips made of dark chocolate, optional

Getting ready:

• Place rolled oats, almond butter, shredded coconut, crushed flaxseeds, honey or maple syrup, and vanilla extract in a big bowl.

• Blend until well blended.

• Form the mixture into balls that are bite-sized.

• You may sprinkle melted dark chocolate over the energy bites if you'd like.

• Before serving, place in the refrigerator for at least half an hour.

Recipe: **Chia Seed and Berry Parfait**

Elements:

• One cup of mixed berries, including raspberries, blueberries, and strawberries

• One cup Greek yoghurt or a substitute made without dairy

• Two tsp full of chia seeds

• One tablespoon agave nectar or honey

• Granola as a garnish

Getting ready:

• In a bowl, combine chia seeds, honey, or agave nectar with Greek yoghurt or a dairy-free substitute.

• To thicken, leave the chia seed mixture in the fridge for at least two hours or overnight.

• Arrange mixed berries on top of the chia seed mixture in serving glasses.

• For extra crunch, sprinkle granola over top.

• Serve cold, tasting the wonderful harmony of flavours and textures.

Recipe: **Apples with Cinnamon Baked**

Elements:

• Four cored and sliced apples

• Two teaspoons of coconut oil, melted

• One tablespoon of maple syrup

• One tsp finely ground cinnamon

• One-quarter tsp nutmeg

• Optional chopped nuts as a garnish

Getting ready:

• Set oven temperature to 375°F, or 190°C.

• Combine apple slices, melted coconut oil, maple syrup, nutmeg, and ground cinnamon in a bowl.

The coated apple slices should be spread out on a baking sheet.

• Bake the apples for 20 to 25 minutes, or until they are soft.

• If preferred, garnish with chopped nuts.

• Serve warm for a soothing and suitable dessert for fibromyalgia.

Concluding Remarkable Balance of Health

These dessert dishes are the epitome of a healthy-yet-indulgent marriage, tailored to the specific dietary needs of fibromyalgia patients. Every dish is an uncompromising celebration of sweet joy, from the rich and velvety Avocado Chocolate Mousse to the healthful deliciousness of Almond Butter Energy Bites and the revitalising Berry and Chia Seed Parfait.

Flavour is not compromised in the realm of fibromyalgia-friendly sweets; rather, it is accentuated by the inherent sweetness of healthful ingredients. Savour the pleasure of these sweets with the knowledge that each mouthful enhances both your pleasure and general health. Chapter 9, as we traverse the territory of fibromyalgia-friendly recipes, is a tribute to the delectable options available to individuals who are looking for sweetness within the parameters of indulgence that is health aware.

Chapter 10: Smoothies and Restorative Drinks

The road towards holistic wellbeing often starts where flavour and sustenance converge. Chapter 10 of "Cooking for Fibromyalgia Wellness" presents a variety of Restorative Beverages and Smoothies that are intended to do more than simply satisfy your thirst; they are also meant to act as comfort elixirs, relieving pain and promoting general wellbeing.

Calming Blends for Fibromyalgia Pain Reduction

When creating these healing drinks, elements with calming and anti-inflammatory qualities are prioritised. The idea is to make beverages that help manage the symptoms of fibromyalgia while also providing a sense of refreshment. These two dishes serve as examples:

Recipe: **Ginger-Turmeric Tea**

Elements:

• One tsp finely ground turmeric

• One tsp freshly grated ginger

• One tsp honey

• Juiced one lemon

• Two cups heated water

Getting ready:

• Place the grated ginger and ground turmeric in a cup.

• Cover the mixture with boiling water and steep for five to seven minutes.

• Include the freshly squeezed lemon juice and honey.

• Enjoy the anti-inflammatory benefits of this golden elixir by giving it a good stir.

Recipe: **Sleep Aid with Cherries and Almonds**

Elements:

• One cup of sweet cherry juice

• One half banana

• 1/4 cup of overnight-soaked almonds

• Half a teaspoon of extract from almonds

• One-third cup chia seeds

• Ice cubes, if desired

Getting ready:

• Put banana, soaked almonds, chia seeds, almond essence, and tart cherry juice in a blender.

• Process until smooth. If you want a cooler consistency, add ice cubes.

• Pour into a glass and enjoy the peaceful taste of cherries and almonds, which are linked to a better night's sleep.

Hydration Drinks for Everyday Well-Being

Maintaining proper hydration is essential for good health, and these delicious hydration infusions are also a great source of vitamins and minerals. Two hydrating recipes are provided here:

Recipe: **Water Infused with Cucumber and Mint**

Elements:

• Half a cucumber, cut thinly

• Newly harvested mint leaves

• One finely sliced lemon

• Two quarts of water

Getting ready:

• In a pitcher, mix cucumber slices, lemon slices, and mint leaves.

• Pour water into the pitcher.

• To enable the flavours to fully develop, refrigerate for a minimum of two hours.

• For a crisp and revitalising sensation, serve over ice.

Recipe: **Fruity and Citrus Electrolyte Cocktail**

Elements:

• One cup of mixed berries, including raspberries, blueberries, and strawberries

• One juiced orange

• One tsp honey

• One-fourth teaspoon sea salt

• Two cups of coconut water

Getting ready:

• Process orange juice, sea salt, honey, and mixed berries until smooth.

If preferred, strain the mixture to get rid of the seeds.

Blend the berry mixture with coconut water to create a tasty, high-electrolyte beverage.

• To keep you hydrated and feeling revitalised, chill and serve over ice.

Smoothies that Invigorate for Vitality

These smoothies are not only tasty but also nutrient-dense, providing you with energy for the day. These two dishes combine a colourful blend of tastes with many health advantages:

Recipe: **Vegetable Power Shake**

Elements:

• One cup of spinach leaves

• Half a cucumber, chopped and peeled

• One cored and sliced green apple

• One-half avocado

• One-third cup chia seeds

• One cup of coconut water

• Ice cubes, if desired

Getting ready:

• Blend together spinach, cucumber, avocado, apple, chia seeds, and coconut water in a blender.

• Blend until creamy and smooth.

• For an even more nutrient-dense and refreshing green smoothie, add ice cubes if preferred and blend once more.

Recipe: **Smoothie with Mango Turmeric Bliss**

Elements:

• One cup of chunky frozen mango

• One half banana

• Half a teaspoon of turmeric powder

• Half a teaspoon grated ginger

• One cup almond milk

• One-third cup flaxseeds

Getting ready:

• Blend together frozen mango chunks, banana, almond milk, flaxseeds, ginger, and turmeric in a blender.

• Blend until creamy and smooth.

• Transfer into a glass and savour the tastes of the tropics along with turmeric's anti-inflammatory properties.

Tailoring for Individual Wellbeing

The versatility of these healing drinks and smoothies is one of their best features. You are welcome to alter the recipes to suit your tastes and any particular health requirements. These recipes are a blank canvas for you to customise to your own path towards health, whether that means playing around with the sweetness levels, trying out new fruits, or adding more nutrients.

The skill of creating healing drinks and smoothies becomes a thoughtful discipline in Chapter 10 of "Cooking for Fibromyalgia Wellness," fusing the holistic benefits of sustenance with the delights of flavour. Accept these mixtures as elixirs of life as well as beverages, bolstering your health while you navigate the road of fibromyalgia.

Chapter 11: A Holistic Wellness Toolbox: Healing Herbs and Spices

When it comes to creating fibromyalgia-friendly recipes, herbs and spices have just as much healing power as actual ingredients. In Chapter 11, this fragrant cosmos is explored, and the therapeutic qualities that may help with fibromyalgia symptoms and overall wellbeing are revealed.

Overview: Disclosing Nature's Pharmacy

Let's first examine the significant effects that some herbs and spices may have on our health before getting into more detail. Spices and herbs are nature's pharmacy, full of chemicals with anti-inflammatory, analgesic, and antioxidant properties that do more than just improve flavour. Including these nutritional powerhouses into your diet becomes a comprehensive approach to wellbeing when it comes to fibromyalgia, where controlling pain and inflammation is essential.

Cooking with Spices and Herbs for Healing

1. Turmeric: The Magical Concoction

Component:

• Ground turmeric or fresh turmeric root

Recipe: **Turmeric Lentil Soup**

Elements:

• 1 cup red lentils, washed

• 1 onion, diced

• 2 carrots, sliced

• 2 cloves garlic, minced

• 1 tablespoon fresh ginger, grated

• One tsp finely ground turmeric

• 1 teaspoon ground cumin

• 1/2 teaspoon ground coriander

• 4 cups vegetable broth

• Season with salt and pepper to taste

• Fresh cilantro for decorating

Getting ready:

• In a saucepan, sauté the onion, garlic, and ginger until softened.

• Add the ground turmeric, cumin, and coriander, stirring to coat the veggies.

• Add the lentils and vegetable broth, bring to a boil, then simmer until the lentils are cooked.

• Season with salt and pepper, and sprinkle with fresh cilantro before serving.

2. Ginger: Vitality for Digestive Well-being

Component:

• Raw ginger root

Recipe: **Infusion of Ginger and Lemongrass Tea**

Elements:

• Slicing one tablespoon of fresh ginger

• One bruised lemongrass stalk

• Two cups of water

• Agave syrup or honey (optional)

Getting ready:

• Bring the water in a saucepan to a boil.

• Include the bruised lemongrass and ginger pieces.

After ten minutes of simmering, pour into cups.

• If preferred, sweeten with agave syrup or honey.

Cinnamon: Delightful Solace for Pain Relief

Component:

• Cinnamon sticks or ground

Recipe: **Baked Apples with Cinnamon**

Elements:

• Four cored and halved apples

• Two tsp pure maple syrup

• One tsp finely ground cinnamon

• 1/4 cup of chopped nuts, either almonds or walnuts

Getting ready:

• Set oven temperature to 375°F, or 190°C.

The apple halves should be put on a baking dish.

• Sprinkle with ground cinnamon and drizzle with maple syrup.

• Bake the apples for 20 to 25 minutes, or until they are soft.

• Before serving, sprinkle chopped nuts over top.

4. Rosemary: Fragrant Joy for Clear Minds

Component:

• Fresh sprigs of rosemary

Recipe: **Roasted Vegetables with Rosemary**

Elements:

• Chop various veggies (carrots, potatoes, bell peppers, etc.).

• Two teaspoons of olive oil

• One tablespoon finely chopped fresh rosemary

• Season with salt and pepper to taste

Getting ready:

Start the oven to 400°F, or 200°C.

• Combine the chopped veggies, fresh rosemary, olive oil, salt, and pepper in a bowl.

After spreading them out on a baking sheet, roast the veggies for 25 to 30 minutes, or until they are soft and golden.

In conclusion, "A Culinary Adventure to Wellbeing"

Herbs and spices have the power to improve health and flavour; Chapter 11 takes you on a tour through this potential. Every recipe is a step towards holistic wellness, whether it's adding turmeric's anti-inflammatory properties to a soup, enjoying the aromatic bliss of rosemary-roasted vegetables, or nursing a soothing ginger and lemongrass tea for digestive health.

When you include these therapeutic herbs and spices into your fibromyalgia-friendly recipes, think of it as a kind of self-care—a prescription for health and well-being via food. Accept the colourful, fragrant world of nature's medicine and learn to love cooking for your health as much as your pleasure. This chapter offers more than simply recipes; it's an invitation to use your kitchen's healing powers and turn every meal into a step towards overall wellbeing on your path to recovery from fibromyalgia.

Chapter 12: Practical Cooking Methods for Fibromyalgia-Friendly Dinners.

Meal preparation may become a reasonable and joyful part of your routine with deliberate planning and useful tools, even if cooking provides special obstacles for those with fibromyalgia. This chapter delves into culinary techniques and kitchen hacks that prioritise fibromyalgia-friendly foods while making cooking easier.

1. Effective Meal Planning:

Meal prep done well is the key to overcoming kitchen weariness. Think about making large quantities of fibromyalgia-friendly staples, such quinoa, roasted veggies, and lean meats, early in the week. This enables you to quickly and easily prepare healthy meals throughout the week by saving time and energy.

Recipe: **Quinoa with Roasted Vegetable Bowls**

Elements:

• Two cups prepared quinoa.

• A variety of veggies, such as cherry tomatoes, zucchini, and bell peppers

• Olive oil

• Pepper and salt

• Optional lemon-tahini dressing

Getting ready:

• Combine salt, pepper, and olive oil with chopped veggies.

• Bake until the food is soft.

• Fill bowls with quinoa, roasted veggies, and dressing made with lemon and tahini.

2. One-Pan Enchantments:

Accept one-pan recipes to expedite your cooking process and simplify cleaning. By using fewer pots and pans, these recipes increase the accessibility of cooking for people with fibromyalgia.

Recipe: **Chicken with Vegetables and Lemon Herbs on a Sheet Pan**

Elements:

• Chicken thighs or breasts

• A variety of veggies, such as potatoes, carrots, and broccoli

• Olive oil

• Juice from lemons

• Fresh herbs (thyme, rosemary)

• Pepper and salt

Getting ready:

• Arrange the veggies and chicken on a sheet pan.

• Add a drizzle of lemon juice and olive oil, then season with salt, pepper, and herbs.

• Roast the chicken until it's well done and the veggies are soft.

3. The Magic of the Slow Cooker:

Your friend when it comes to making tender, flavorful meals with little effort on your part is the slow cooker. It's an amazing tool for making meals that need to simmer for a long time and are suitable for those with fibromyalgia.

Recipe: **Vegetable and Lentil Stew**

Elements:

• One cup of lentils, dried

• Various veggies, such as onions, celery, and carrots

• Broth made with vegetables

• Tomatoes in cans

• Minced garlic

• Salt, pepper, paprika, and cumin

Getting ready:

• Fill the slow cooker with all of the ingredients.

• Simmer for 6 to 8 hours on low.

• Savour a filling and substantial lentil stew.

4. Cooking in batches:

Accept the idea of preparing in bulk so you may accumulate a variety of reheatable, fibromyalgia-friendly foods. This technique is particularly helpful on days when there is a lot of weariness.

Recipe: **Curry with spinach and chickpeas**.

Elements:

• Two drained cans of chickpeas

• Ripe spinach

• Milk from coconuts

• Powdered or paste curry

• Garlic, ginger, and onions

• Rice, basmati (optional)

Getting ready:

• Saute the ginger, garlic, and onions.

• Include the curry spice, spinach, coconut milk, and chickpeas.

• If wanted, serve over rice once the flavours have had time to blend.

5. Carefully Choose Your Ingredients:

Choose fibromyalgia-friendly foods that focus nutrition without sacrificing on flavour. Opt for fresh, natural foods, and experiment with herbs and spices for extra taste without depending excessively on salt or manufactured flavours.

Recipe: **Herb-Infused Baked Salmon**

Elements:

• Salmon fillets

• Fresh herbs (dill, parsley, chives)

• Lemon slices

• Olive oil

• Pepper and salt

Getting ready:

• Place fish on a baking sheet.

• Drizzle with olive oil, sprinkle with chopped herbs, and add lemon slices.

• Bake until the fish is cooked through and flakes easily.

6. Smart Storage Solutions:

Invest in smart storage solutions to keep your kitchen tidy and make meals more efficient. Label and store ready ingredients in transparent containers for easy access, and use freezer-friendly containers for batch-cooked meals.

Example: Mason Jar Salads

Components (arranged in a jar):

• Dressing (such as balsamic vinaigrette) at the bottom layer

• Hard veggies (cucumbers, cherry tomatoes, etc.) are the next layer.

• Proteins or grains (quinoa, grilled chicken, etc.) in the middle layer

• Leafy greens (such as spinach and rocket) at the top layer

Getting ready:

• Put the ingredients in a mason jar according to the suggested sequence.

• Refrigerate after sealing the container.

• For a quick and fresh salad, shake before serving.

7. Innovative Cooking Utensils:

Invest in kitchen appliances that facilitate cooking and lessen stress. You may greatly enhance your cooking experience by using anti-fatigue mats, jar openers, and ergonomic tools.

Recipe: **Zucchini Noodle Spiralizer**

Elements:

• Zucchini

• Olive oil

• Minced garlic

• Tomatillos

• Finely chopped basil

• Cheese Parmesan (optional)

Getting ready:

• Turn courgette spirals into noodles.

• Add the zucchini noodles and simmer until soft after sautéing the garlic in olive oil.

• For a fast and fibromyalgia-friendly spaghetti substitute, top with cherry tomatoes, basil, and Parmesan cheese.

Adding these useful cooking methods and recipes to your repertoire not only makes cooking easier, but it also guarantees that each meal is prepared in accordance with fibromyalgia-friendly nutritional guidelines. You may enjoy tasty, nutritious meals without compromising your health by making wise decisions in the kitchen. Recall that the goal of creating a fibromyalgia-friendly diet is to achieve balance and pleasure in every meal.

Chapter 13: Planning Meals and Including a Lifestyle

For those navigating the terrain of fibromyalgia, Chapter 13 of "Cooking Green: The Ultimate Beginner's Vegetarian Cookbook" becomes a compass in the dynamic fabric of our lives, where health and well-being are interwoven with everyday routines. This chapter goes beyond the kitchen, providing insightful advice on how to create a proactive meal planning strategy for continued nutritional support and health enhancement as well as how to include fibromyalgia-friendly foods into everyday activities.

Meal Planning: An All-encompassing Method

Meal planning is a comprehensive approach to nourishing the body and mind, not simply a matter of choosing what to eat. We take a proactive approach to meal planning in this chapter, understanding that a well-planned menu may help manage the symptoms of fibromyalgia and improve general health.

Example 1: Weekly Balanced Menu

Monday:

• Quinoa salad with roasted vegetables and chickpeas for lunch

• Steamed asparagus and baked lemon herb tilapia for dinner

Wednesday

• Stuffed bell peppers with spinach and feta for lunch.

• Brown rice with lentil and vegetable curry for dinner

This Friday:

• Greek couscous salad with hummus for lunch

• Quinoa Pilaf with Grilled Tofu Skewers for dinner

This plan offers a harmony of tastes, textures, and vital nutrients by sprinkling in a range of nutrient-dense foods throughout the week.

Effective Grocery Buying for Achievement

A well equipped kitchen is the cornerstone of an effective meal plan. This chapter explores effective grocery shopping techniques that assist fibromyalgia sufferers reduce their level of stress and expedite the process of locating foods that are suitable for them.

Example 2: A Grocery List Adapted to Fibromyalgia

• Fresh Vegetables:

• Leafy greens (kale, spinach)

• Vibrant veggies, such as cherry tomatoes and bell peppers

• Fresh herbs (cilantro, parsley)

• Proteins:

• Lean proteins (fish, tofu, and chicken).

• Legumes (lentils, chickpeas)

• Whole Grains:

• Whole-grain couscous, brown rice, and quinoa

• Dairy Substitutes:

• Almond and soy-based plant-based milk

• Yoghurt without dairy

• Good Fats:

• Nuts, avocado, and olive oil

• Herbs & Spices:

• Ginger, cinnamon, and turmeric

When someone has a well thought-out shopping list, they can shop with purpose and make sure they have everything they need for a week's worth of fibromyalgia-friendly meals.

Methods of Preparation for Effectiveness

Given that fibromyalgia may cause difficulties in the kitchen, this chapter offers useful preparatory methods to make cooking easier. These techniques, which range from batch cooking to clever storage options, are meant to make meal preparation easier and more fun.

Example 3: Convenient Batch Cooking

Recipe: **Vegetable Medley with Roasts**:

Elements:

• A variety of veggies, including cherry tomatoes, bell peppers, and zucchini

• Sea salt, pepper, and olive oil

• Getting ready:

Start the oven to 400°F, or 200°C.

• Dice veggies into small pieces.

• Combine salt, pepper, and olive oil.

• After spreading, roast for 20 to 25 minutes on a baking sheet.

• Let cool completely before dividing into servings.

This reduces the need for substantial daily cooking by preparing flexible foods that can be used in a variety of meals throughout the week.

Creating a Kitchen Environment That Is Fibromyalgia-Friendly

This chapter goes beyond the dos and don'ts of meal planning to explore setting up a kitchen that helps people with fibromyalgia. The aim is to make the kitchen a comfortable and joyful place to cook, from ergonomic appliances to organising advice.

Example 4: Kitchen Renovations That Are Fibromyalgia-Friendly

• Ergonomic Implements:

To reduce strain, get tools with comfortable handles.

• To meet various demands, think about getting a cutting board with an adjustable height.

• Solutions for Organisations:

• To make ingredients easily visible, use transparent containers.

• To cut down on bending and reaching, place commonly used things in convenient locations.

People may design a kitchen that suits their own demands by carefully altering the layout, which will improve their cooking experience.

Including Meals That Are Fibromyalgia-Friendly in Everyday Routines

This chapter takes readers from planning to execution, showing them how to easily include fibromyalgia-friendly foods into everyday activities. The emphasis is on developing routines that support general well-being, such as mindful mealtimes and basic rituals.

Example 5: Intentional Mealtime Practice

• Establish a Calm Space:

• When selecting dining linens, choose for calming hues.

• During eating, play relaxing music or natural noises.

• Make Mindful Food Choices:

• Savour each taste with little nibbles.

• Store electrical gadgets to reduce distractions.

People may improve digestion and their entire eating experience by bringing mindfulness into their mealtimes.

In summary, a blueprint for long-term health

Chapter 13 provides a step-by-step guide for incorporating fibromyalgia-friendly foods into everyday living. Every element, from proactive meal planning to effective grocery shopping and preparation methods, is thoughtfully designed to provide the groundwork for long-term health improvement. People with fibromyalgia may confidently manage their culinary journey and transform every meal into a time of pleasure and nutrition by adopting this all-inclusive approach.

DAILY MEAL PLANNER

DAY/DATE: _______________________________

BREAKFAST

GROCERY LIST

LUNCH

DINNER

SNACKS

NOTES

DAILY MEAL PLANNER

DAY/DATE: _______________________________

BREAKFAST

LUNCH

DINNER

SNACKS

GROCERY LIST

NOTES

DAILY MEAL PLANNER

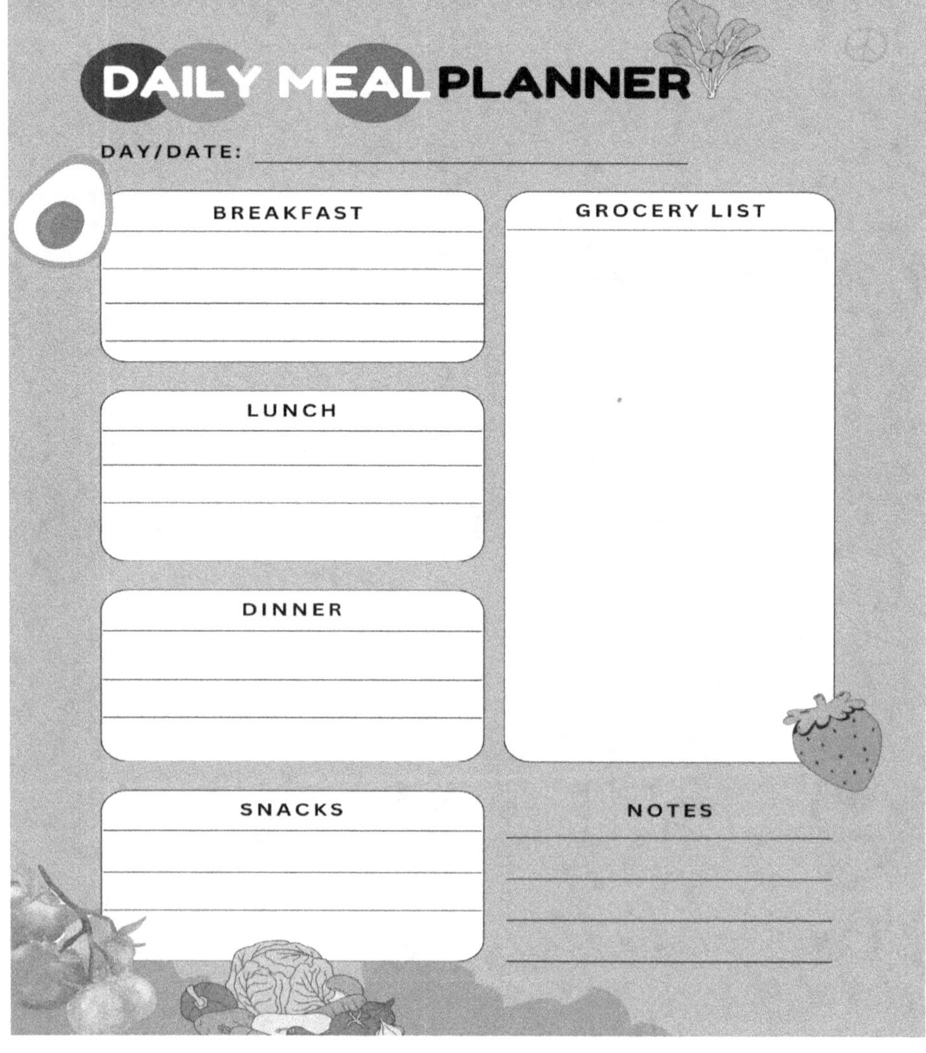

DAY/DATE: ___________________________

BREAKFAST

LUNCH

DINNER

SNACKS

GROCERY LIST

NOTES

DAILY MEAL PLANNER

DAY/DATE: _______________________________

BREAKFAST

LUNCH

DINNER

SNACKS

GROCERY LIST

NOTES

DAILY MEAL PLANNER

DAY/DATE: _______________________

BREAKFAST

GROCERY LIST

LUNCH

DINNER

SNACKS

NOTES

DAILY MEAL PLANNER

DAY/DATE: _______________________________

BREAKFAST

GROCERY LIST

LUNCH

DINNER

SNACKS

NOTES

DAILY MEAL PLANNER

DAY/DATE: ______________________

BREAKFAST

LUNCH

DINNER

SNACKS

GROCERY LIST

NOTES

DAILY MEAL PLANNER

DAY/DATE: _______________________________

BREAKFAST

GROCERY LIST

LUNCH

DINNER

SNACKS

NOTES